Post Trauma
and
Chronic
Emotional Fatigue

By Billie J. Sahley, Ph.D., C.N.C.

Pain & Stress Publications®
San Antonio, Texas
October 2002

Note to Readers

This material is not intended to replace the services of a physician, nor is it meant to encourage diagnosis and treatment of illness, disease, or other medical problems by the layman. This book should not be regarded as a substitute for professional medical treatment and while every care is taken to ensure the accuracy of the content, the author and the publishers cannot accept legal responsibility for any problem arising out of experimentation with the methods described. Any application of the recommendations set forth in the following pages is at the reader's discretion and sole risk. If you are under a physician's care for any condition, he or she can advise you as to whether the program described in this book is suitable for you.

No part of this publication may be reproduced, stored in a retrieval system, or transmitted in any form or by any means, electronic, mechanical, photocopying, recording, or otherwise, without the prior written permission of the author.

This publication has been compiled through research resources at the Pain & Stress Center, San Antonio, TX 78229.

1st Edition, 1994
2nd Edition, October 1995
3rd Edition, October 2002

Printed in U.S.A.
Additional copies may be ordered from:
Pain & Stress Center
5282 Medical Drive, Suite 160, San Antonio, Texas 78229-6023

1-800-669-2256 or
Visit our web site: http://www.painstresscenter.com

ISBN 1-889391-21-2
Library of Congress# 2002110220

Dedication

My associates and staff whose timeless help and support gave me the precious time for the research and writing.

To the Lord for always lighting my path.

Contents

Introduction

All too often, when a patient with post trauma stress and chronic emotional fatigue goes to a physician to find out what is wrong, the patient will be told he might have post trauma stress, chronic fatigue, or depression. This book is to help those who suffer from post trauma stress and chronic emotional fatigue to understand it and conquer it. It is not meant to pass judgments on what you are feeling and why.

Post trauma and chronic emotional fatigue do in many ways mimic chronic fatigue but that is where it ends. In *Harrison's Principles of Internal Medicine*, it states 50 to 80 % of all disease is psychosomatic in nature. This means there is no pathology or disease involved in most illnesses. This does not mean there's not pain, there is, a lot of it!

The key is that chronic emotional fatigue is stress induced. Post trauma and chronic emotional fatigue result from a traumatic episode or experience that you have no control over or from an accident, loss of a loved one, a divorce, or any event that causes prolonged uncertainty and stress. Caregivers to a loved one who passes on after a long-term illness are lost in grief and depression and feel they will never heal. The mind becomes so saturated that the mental stress surfaces as physical symptoms, a little at first, then a constant flow. The immune system breaks down, fatigue sets in as well as depression, fear, anxiety, and uncertainty.

To my knowledge, there has not been any research published on post trauma and chronic emotional fatigue. I published the first information on chronic emotional fatigue in 1992. Chronic emotional fatigue and post traumatic stress affect millions of people who have been searching for answers to their many health problems. I plan to continue my research in this area and to update my findings, as information becomes available in future publications.

As you read the information in this book, let your healing begin!

Billie J. Sahley, Ph.D., C.N.C.

Recognizing Post Trauma and Chronic Emotional Fatigue

Millions of people suffer from post trauma and chronic emotional fatigue (CEF) and their greatest <u>fear</u> is that they will never recover from it. They live in a constant state of anxiety because they do not understand exactly what their problem is. Post trauma and chronic emotional fatigue are curable. Understanding the symptoms and their causes is the first step of healing. Post traumatic stress and chronic emotional fatigue act in very subtle ways and can come on gradually and insidiously. Few people recognize the problems or know that the many symptoms they dread are no more than the symptoms of constant, unrelenting stress that leads to post trauma and chronic emotional fatigue.

Let me explain the anatomy of post trauma and chronic emotional fatigue, how it works, how you can cope with it, and even conquer it. The more you understand about your symptoms, the less stress, anxiety, and fear can control you. The information in this book is based on years of research, patient observations, and interviews.

Post trauma and chronic emotional fatigue are an overload of sensory information to the limbic system in the brain, especially the amygdala. The limbic system is known as the feelings part of the brain; it regulates emotions. The amygdala is the brain's alarm system. The amygdala is where experiences are stored for later playback. Traumatic or stressful events are released via the amygdala and cause the extreme feelings of fear, panic, and hopelessness. The amygdala provides a subconscious rating of intensity to every stimulus you address, even before you are aware of it.

The amygdala is a small pea-shaped pod in front of the brain that responds to everything and gives an emotional tag for future reference and response. Any emotional overlap can intensify the symptoms of chronic emotional fatigue such as physical fatigue. By that, I mean bodily weariness, or it can surface as anxious fatigue or mental fatigue, the type of fatigue that affects the mind. This fatigue seems to rob the sufferer of the will to get better. Because of the complex natures of chronic emotional fatigue and chronic stress syndrome, patients must understand how their brain and body store emotions.

Emotions are simultaneously everywhere in the body. Emotions and stress-related thoughts always move in an upward direction, which increases or causes more anxiety often after an emotional experience. CEF and chronic stress syndrome do not happen overnight. They accumulate over months or even years from nonstop fatigue and stress exhaustion. Post trauma, CEF, and chronic stress syndrome brings about an intense, nagging, painful loss of control that affects every nerve fiber in your brain and body. Few people recognize it or know that the many symptoms they dread are no more than the symptoms of the constant, unrelenting stress and anxiety that lead to full-blown emotional fatigue. However, the knowledge and understanding of what is happening to you is a very powerful healer. Healing is the key. This thought must take over your thinking process so the brain programs it. Do not be impatient! Time, knowledge, and healing will gradually recharge your batteries, especially after the age of 40.

Ordinarily, physical fatigue is easy enough to recognize. Fatigue comes to everyone after strenuous exercise, playing tennis, or walking five miles. It feels good after a hot shower or hot tub to lie in bed tired but relaxed and even enjoy the feeling of aching muscles. But the physical fatigue that comes with anxious fatigue is not enjoyable. It does not come from the extra use of muscles. It comes from the abuse of muscles by subjecting them to the tension that accompanies constant anxiety, stress, and post trauma.

Resting muscles are in the condition called tone and are firm and ready for action, not limp or weak. They are kept in tone by reflex nervous action. You probably know what reflex action is. If I were to tap your knee just below your kneecap, your leg would jerk automatically. That is reflex action. I could make your leg jerk this way all day without making you become tired. However, tension uses nervous energy, and it allows the chemicals of muscular fatigue such as lactic acid to collect within the muscles and bloodstream. This is why an anxious and stressed person so often complains of aching legs, back, and neck. This kind of ache is so constant that if you are anxious and had to stand for a few minutes, you would look around for some place to sit or head straight home to bed where you feel safe.

Later, I'll explain the nutrient deficiencies that cause restless legs and constant muscle spasms. Chronic emotional fatigue is especially puzzling because the sufferer knows it can strike at any time. You want to believe there must be something physically wrong with you. You live in the doctor's office having one test after another. You are even more puzzled because you feel you are almost unable to drag your body out of the bed in the morning. By evening, you may not feel so bad and even feel some improvement. In these moments of relief from suffering, you can sense hope and glimpse the possibility of getting better. You hold onto these times and fear you will lose them. You <u>fear</u> going to bed because you know from experience that morning brings new anxiety, despair, and a weary body—a tiredness almost beyond tiredness with extreme depression.

This is difficult to explain to a family. A patient's husband said to his wife, Louise, "You cannot be tired, you have not done anything all day." Louise said, "Doctor, I can hardly crawl around, and my eyes feel as though they are being dragged out of their sockets. I sit and try to accept. I keep having anxiety attacks. I listen to relaxation tapes, and I try to relax. But my body stays all tied up in spasms something terrible. What am I doing? What's wrong?"

Actually, Louise was not doing what I had told her. Louise was neglecting to take the needed nutrients and amino acids, and she was not practicing her deep breathing to relax. She would spend a few minutes trying to relax and then an hour anxiously waiting to see if her body got the message. I told her to begin walking. Her husband who was listening on the extension phone said, "I have not forced her to do anything."

But if this particular woman were to wait until she felt like walking, she would still be waiting. It is difficult for a person with chronic emotional fatigue and traumatic stress to decide how much work or play they can do without harming themselves. Louise would stand with a paintbrush posed wondering, "Should I really be doing this? Will I get better quicker if I rested? Am I overdoing it?"

The word, *rested*, holds the key to the puzzle. How much does a person with post trauma and chronic emotional fatigue rest when she sits doing nothing? Very little! If a patient like Louise would lie down during the day and try to sleep, her mind would release only negative thinking. With her head on her pillow, it is almost as if she would focus only on how bad she felt. With so much time to concentrate on all the negatives, she becomes more anxious and tense. If she has a problem to worry about, which she always has, by the time she has spent an hour or more concentrating on it, with fear well at work, the problem becomes a major crisis. You can bet it will be health related. She felt more exhausted when she got up than when she first laid down. From then on, she probably will avoid lying down during the day. Uncertainty is the only thought!

If you suffer from emotional fatigue, you may well ask, "Well, how much can I do?" You can attempt anything you feel up to and want to do. I said attempt because I do not want you to set a high standard of achievement. Be satisfied with what little you can do at first. It is the *attempt* that matters. I do not mean that you should paint your house then rush inside for a soft drink and watch television. I mean at least do some work. But, if necessary, do it at a slow pace. As you become more confident that you do not loose control, you may even become interested in what you are doing. Now is when you can really rest. With interest and confidence aroused, the battle is half over. Confidence and interest are tension and anxiety's worst enemies and therefore the enemy of fatigue. A nervously ill person may only have to move quickly to feel the heart, as one man expressed it, "Pound so hard I felt it in my mouth." This is perhaps one of the fearful experiences in post trauma and emotional fatigue. The heart may also, as the layman says, skip beats. If you have been examined by a doctor and told that your symptoms are caused by stress and anxiety, and there is nothing wrong with your heart, do not be upset by your heart's objection to work. Just keep on slowly, and let your muscles get used to being used gradually and released naturally. Just take one day at a time.

Anyone who has been sitting at a desk for months getting little physical exercise will find that his heart will race with little effort, even skip beats. No doctor would suggest that you should keep sitting at your desk and not exercise for fear of damaging your heart. Graduated exercise would be the prescription for you, just as it is for the emotionally fatigued or stressed person—racing heart or no racing heart. A good massage will help sore, aching muscles and do worlds of good. Lack of confidence keeps so many people wrapped up in fear and anxiety.

Some years ago I persuaded a patient, Glen, to go swimming. Glen thought he would get so exhausted that he would not be able to walk the distance to the beach. Yet, he managed to do so and then stood shivering with anxiety at the edge of the water. Glen was sure he would have a heart attack when he walked into the water. If he could hardly manage to walk the fifty yards to the beach, how could he find the strength to swim? Finally, with the fear, Glen entered the water not only fearing the worst but now prepared for it, muscles tensed. But as he began to swim, the memory of all those other occasions when he swam well brought him a little confidence. For once, past memory was his friend instead of his foe playing old tapes of fear. After a little while, he struck out into deeper water. He was actually enjoying swimming. I heard no more about the stress and anxiety of walking home.

In one daring exercise, Glen gained more confidence and felt more strength than if he had rested for weeks. I hope you are getting my message. Relax; do not fear everything you do will cause you pain. That thought alone wears you out and takes all your energy. You will be tired for days because of the *"what if"* fear. The problem of chronic emotional fatigue, stress, and post trauma began with *what if, what if, and what if!*

A person who suffers from post traumatic stress and chronic emotional fatigue has anxiety and panic that zaps every drop of energy that they have. *That is why I say challenge yourself daily.* Women are especially bad. The whole day is an effort. She probably has to take her children to school each morning, drive home, do the housework, wash, shop, pick up the children after school, cook dinner, bath the children and get them to bed. If you are reading this hoping that I have a magic bullet for you, I must break the news; I do not! The only magic lies in your attitude toward the situation. You must be prepared to work slowly at a pace you can manage. If that means crawling, then you must crawl and not blame yourself for working this way. Do not blame yourself because of how you feel. You think you are letting your family down. Do not blame yourself if you do not clean the house or if the meals are not as satisfactory as you think they should be. Do not knock yourself too often for letting a neighbor pick up the children after school.

If you are like this woman, you should try to put yourself into neutral. Back off, relax, and take time to enjoy the day. Do not make demands on yourself. Go to your own corner of the world—a place where you feel safe and no one can bother you. It means setting no standards at this stage. Above all, you must go forward as willingly as you can manage. Willingness relieves tension and also fatigue. And by willingly, I really mean willingly do everything. Rest willingly and accept overtiredness willingly. If you cannot decide how much you should do and seem to sit wondering, accept this willingly. Accept everything willingly and stop fighting the rain. Above all, close the door on self-pity, and spoil yourself a little. In my first book, *The Anxiety Epidemic,* I call this *taking time to smell the flowers*—it is a good phrase, remember it. Steal a few minutes of enjoyment for yourself. Buy a book you want and read it. If the clothes need ironing, allow yourself rest periods during the day. Even if the ceiling is cracking and threatens to fall, give yourself permission to relax a few minutes. When I am working hard, especially writing for hours, at the end of each hour, whether I am tired or not, I sit back for five minutes. I take several deep breaths and go to my little corner of the world so my shoulders rest and relax. I get the rest in before the pain begins. Stay relaxed, and you will be more productive. Remember, deep breathing alone changes your brain chemistry and increases neurotransmitters.

Many patients with post trauma and chronic emotional fatigue ask if they should continue to work. My answer is yes. If you have post trauma, stress, and chronic emotional fatigue, many problems can arise if you do not have an employer who understands or is not sensitive to your problem. Since no two people are alike, each must be advised individually. You and your employer should consider the work problems and levels of stress. If you feel work is stressful, try to figure out why. Then talk it out and make positive changes. Do not withdraw and get depressed.

Emotional fatigue depends a great deal on just how sensitized a person's nerves are. To test yourself, try this experiment to illustrate the meaning of sensitization. Sit in a room with soft music and dim lights and notice how relaxing it is. Then turn up the lights and change the station to hip-hop or loud hard rock music. Notice that your breathing changes, your muscles contract, and you become nervous and edgy. This demonstrates how your nerves become oversensitized due to loud noise, bright lights, and uncertainty. If the amygdala is hypersensitive, research shows it results in anxiety, post trauma, and panic. Sensitized nerves make a very sensitive sounding board. There is nothing wrong with your nerves. They are simply responding to constant hammering by anxiety, tension, fear, and uncertainty.

Sensitized nerves register emotion in an exaggerated way. This is difficult for an emotionally fatigued person to understand and deal with. You may feel a mild dislike transgressing into intolerance where a few minutes waiting seems like hours and soft music becomes loud noise. The simple tap of a spoon against a saucer reverberates painfully on overly sensitized ears. A child's crying sends an anxious, stressed, or emotionally fatigued person searching for dark solitude. So over sensitized, the sight of someone you love brings tears and a rare minute of joy may be felt hysterically. A person in this state feels buffeted by an unknown force as though they swing up and down on an emotional swing. Many patients feel they will never have energy and enjoy life with family and friends as they once did.

Living with exaggerated emotions requires much energy. Emotional reserves can eventually be so drained that you becomes apathetic, then depressed. It is not easy to understand that when you are apathetic, you may have little emotional reserve to handle ordinary everyday feelings. You may no longer feel love for your spouse or family. An empty spot exists where feelings used to be and even interest in sex diminishes.

Although post trauma and chronic emotional fatigue sufferers feel like this, they always manage to find enough reserve to register anxiety, fear, and panic. Chronic emotional stress and fatigue are very bewildering as they cut a hole right through the middle of your life. You can lose all hope and feel totally helpless. When you understand sensitization and the feeling it brings, the myths begin to clear. Things have meaning. Fear and uncertainty do not direct your life.

Severe chronic emotional fatigue and depression go hand

in hand. You should think of depression as depletion of the mind and body. Depression implies a downward direction—a depth out of which the depressed person must somehow drag himself. Most feel it is an endless struggle, but it does not have to be. You can clear yourself not only of depression that is depletion but also chronic stress and fatigue. Stop struggling and start healing. The healing will be gradual, but it will happen. Blaming everybody and everything will not get you out of depression. Rather, it makes you feel more tired and depleted. Go out and meet people and keep busy. Too often, you feel better when you are out and become depressed as soon as you see your home. Why? You begin playing old tapes because you are surrounded by old memories, old pain, and habits. Solving the mystery of traumatic stress and fatigue is a task that is yours alone.

Please remember, recovery and healing from stress, trauma, and fatigue will be gradual. You have been running on empty for a long time and dipped deeply into emotional reserves. It will take time for these reserves to be replenished— to balance your brain chemistry and re-educate your muscles to activity. Each emotion must run its course, and each loss must bear its hurt. Patience is the key. Prepare yourself to work through your feelings of depression. You need to be in a place of acceptance. What has happened has happened; it is not happening now, so do not let it take control of your life. Let it go, and let today be the first day of the rest of your life. The difference between a happy life and an unhappy one is the way you come to terms with accepting pain and loss.

Please remember recovery from depletion is gradual just as it takes time for a wound to heal. You must work with your feelings of depression. Leave the depression in the past to enjoy the present. Do not allow depression to control your thinking or healing progress.

If your doctor suggests antidepressants, they are not an answer; they will not help. Tell your doctor you prefer using a natural alternative such as amino acids. Amino acids treat the problem, not just the symptoms. Behavior and orthomolecular therapists and doctors know how to treat post traumatic stress and chronic emotional fatigue. Your immune system must be restored and your brain chemistry put back into balance. I devoted a complete section at the end of this book to help you with an orthomolecular approach.

Case Studies

Rosemary was a forty-three year old mother of two who had gone through a traumatic experience and had problems with depression. During one of our sessions she told me that some of her friends were trying to convince her that taking antidepressants was an answer. I told Rosemary no chronically stressed or fatigued person should be tied to taking antidepressants! I explained to her that a depressed, chronically fatigued person would recover without antidepressants. I have never suggested them, and all of my patients are doing well. According to Peter Breggin, M.D., in his book *Toxic Psychiatry*, it makes no sense to give toxic drugs that impair brain function.

If you are willing to work on the understanding that feelings of depression are a form of depletion, the temporary symptoms will soon pass. Time and healing will gradually recharge your batteries, especially after the age of forty. Do not become impatient! Above all, beware of another draining emotion, despair. Despair can carry your spirits down a doom and gloom cycle and prolong healing.

Jan, a thirty-six year old teacher suffering from chronic emotional fatigue lost a close friend to cancer. Jan asked me what she should do about the funeral in her present state of mind. I advised her to do what she felt she could handle. The only expectations she had to live up to were her own. Grief and emotional fatigue make you feel overwhelmed by even the smallest things, let alone the death of a friend. She went to the funeral and sat in the back. She did not view her friend as she chose to remember her as she was when she was alive, not as she was in the coffin. Halfway through the service, she left.

Later, Jan told me she felt like a failure. She was not a failure. She was only protecting her already over-sensitized nervous system. Sometimes an incident of this nature brings on feelings of guilt that become very intense and deeply hurts the sensitized person that feels they will never recover. Feelings of guilt must be dealt with one at a time until they diminish. Be careful not to let guilt open old wounds because your mind and body have reached a point of saturation. Do not play old tapes! Let the past stay in the past!

Acceptance, obviously, may not carry you upwards, but it does stop you from sinking into despair. As I already mentioned, finding something interesting to do, especially with other people, does help. It is very difficult for a homemaker going through the daily chores to find interest. Her main hope is to accept depletion as willingly as she can. Working with it, knowing that if she does, it will also allow her to feel better sooner. Your emotions are who you are.

Brain fatigue is mental fatigue. Constant anxious, inward thinking in post traumatic stress and chronic emotional fatigue brings brain drain that, of course, is mental fatigue. Thoughts slow down and thinking becomes an effort instead of thoughts flitting lightly from subject to subject as they do when you are fresh. In a chronically, emotionally drained or stressed person thoughts come with a great deal of effort. It is almost as if each thought has to be worked through twice. These sufferers become easily confused, finding concentration and remembering arduous. Talking to others becomes such a strain that when the chronically tired or stressed person sees a neighbor approaching, they cross to the other side of the street to avoid them. Similarly, they avoid answering the telephone like the plague. Before they were ill, they spent hours on the weekend sitting in the sun, lazily dipping into the newspaper, sometimes hardly thinking at all. Time spent now drags by minute by minute. Thoughts that come slowly seem difficult to discard. It is almost as if they stick in the mind.

This is one reason why a mentally tired person gnaws at a problem and seems unable to let it go. One woman said that although she knew she loved her husband, the thought that she did not, kept recurring. The thoughts were so convincing, she began to think they must be true. I explained that the thoughts were convincing her because she was sensitized, and therefore, it made such a deep impression. I also explained that the thoughts kept returning because she was going back to them.

In chronic emotional fatigue and stress, fear works by throwing off frightening ideas that may seem impossible. Never be disturbed by this. Never fight to release an unwanted thought. Let it come. Take it with you. Work with it. Resolve it and let it go. If you fight, you only add more tension, and you make the thought seem more important than it is. Once you make it important, it is much more difficult to forget. You should not fight to forget it. You make it unimportant by taking it with you. See it for what it is, only a thought. Work with it. It will soon dissolve with time as though it was never there.

Joan, a menopausal patient in her fifties disclosed she had

reoccurring thoughts that she did not love her husband. The thought seemed to come when she was very tired and mentally depleted. Joan described them as forceful and clinging, almost demanding her attention. Then when she was able to put everything into perspective, she could see it for what it was, only a thought. When she related it, it seemed so silly, and she could even smile at it, especially when we broke it down in therapy.

I call this sudden fleeting ability to see distressing thoughts in true prospective, realistic observation. The chronically stressed and emotionally fatigued person may be able to observe the truth, or perhaps even another acceptable point of view, only once or twice daily. But that brief observation is enough to show them the trick mental fatigue is playing on them. It is enough to encourage a person not to take upsetting ideas too seriously at this stage of healing. Also, with mental tiredness, forgetting becomes a problem; you begin to believe you have Attention Deficit Disorder (ADD). But, you do not!

Another patient named Carla said, "Doctor, you would not believe the terrible thoughts that keep bugging me, unreal thoughts." Of course, I believed her. I have heard about such thoughts often. If you cannot remember, leave notes for yourself, and if you forget where you put the notes, see the humor in it. Does it matter so much whether you remember now? You *will* remember only too easily when you are well. You remember things you would rather forget. Forgetting easily is all part of emotional fatigue and trauma. An anxious person worries continually about the state he is in. He gradually loses interest in other things, and the outside world may become unreal.

Feelings of unreality are what you make of them, and they are always an offshoot of fear or anxiety. Feeling unreal does not mean you are going crazy, nor does it mean you are permanently losing touch with the world. You have been fearful about your illness for so long that thinking about it seems more natural than thinking about other things. Feel as unreal as you want to, just do not be frightened by it. I promise you that when you begin to recover, other interests return, and the feelings of unreality fade, like a cloudy day.

Fatigue can accentuate unreality. This sets off a chain reaction of unreal feelings and your fear intensifies. If your vision is blurred, you fear you have a disease in your eyes. You start a worry pattern. This pattern influences your behavior and your will to heal and live pain and stress free.

Dr. Carolyn Myss in her book *Why People Don't Heal* outlines how every illness we have corresponds to a pattern of psychological stresses, beliefs, and attitudes that influence corresponding areas of the body. Dr. Myss's research follows the exact philosophy as Dr. Kenneth Pelletier's book *Mind as Healer, Mind as Slayer* that establishes the relationship between mental stress and physical symptoms. Can you see how important understanding is and how intense stress and anxiety can trick you into believing you will never heal? Stress affects every organ in your body, and yes, it can even blur your vision just as it can make your heart race and your hands tremble. Again, acceptance is the key. *Stay in reality and stay relaxed.*

Fatigue of belief is directed at the chronic pain, stress, and anxiety that control your life. Maybe you feel the struggle has been too much and you loose the will to heal. Many patients tell me they feel old, tired, and brain drained. They cannot bear the thought of thinking about the future. The thought of facing tomorrow and believing they will heal is almost beyond them. But healing and changing your belief holds the key to a bright future. You will go through many transitions before you reach your goal. If you feel fatigue of belief, you have identified a major stressor that feeds post traumatic stress and chronic emotional fatigue. The key to coping is stop struggling against the feelings of stress, anxiety, and fatigue; the more you struggle to avoid them, the more anxious, fatigued, and fearful you become. I know it is not easy to relax and go forward into the uncertainty that the symptoms bring. It is not easy to work with an unknown future. This is classic anticipatory fear; it causes the brain to unleash a release of adrenaline and cortisol into the bloodstream setting up the *fight-or-flight* response. The response is supposed to be a short-lived reaction, yet today most of us are in and out of this state continually due to the chronic stress and anxiety. Homeostasis is the key to protect your immune system from further damage while your healing journey continues.

If you have had only some of these experiences I have been talking about, do not immediately become upset and think, "Does all that have to happen to me?" It does not. By implementing what I have explained, you will understand and have some idea of how to cope with emotional fatigue. The key to coping is stop struggling. When you struggle against the feelings, you become more tense, more fatigued, more sensitized, more anxious, and more fearful. So stop struggling.

A mother loved her daughter dearly but dreaded her coming home on weekends. She shuttered from the thought of having to listen to a million questions and the daughter's critical gaze as she asked hopefully, "Are you any better, Mother?" Then her depression started, and she would go back to point A.

Recently this woman telephoned to say that the morning had been especially rough for her. But she came through it by saying to herself, "I will feel better in an hour or so." I will listen to a relaxation tape and do slow, deep breathing until I feel relaxed and in control. I will have some peace then, and my body will relax. The thought of peace to come sustained her. But while she lived for those peaceful moments, she made very little progress. I explained that true lasting peace did not lie in the moments of relief from suffering. These were only rest periods or intermissions. The real peace lay deep within her and cried to come out.

The peace would be reflected in her attitudes at the time when she was feeling the dreaded sensations at their peak. That was the moment when she had to find real peace through acceptance of the symptoms by not struggling and being willing to work with her feelings. She thought for a while and then said, "You mean I have to find the eye of the storm." She had the right message at last. Sailors say that at the center of a storm, there is a place of peace that they call the "eye." The storm swirls around it, but you cannot touch it. If you are to find it, you must first sail through the storm. If that woman would work as willingly as possible with the storm raging, she would find the eye of the storm within herself. She would have found real peace, although the symptoms were still present. True peace lies not in the absence of symptoms, but close by. When you have found this peace, you will eventually find the other peace—the peace that comes when the symptoms have finally gone and your healing is in progress.

The next day, the woman reported that while in pain, she sat at work. She was a writer and worked for two hours, and for the first time in years, she was able to almost lose herself in the work while the storm raged. Somehow the storm did not seem so important. It takes courage to go into the storm. It is more usual to think that you must hold on. If you do not, the symptoms get worse. That woman had been holding on for years without relief. Is it not time she tried letting go? Try going into the storm willingly or as willingly as you can manage.

I want you to practice willingness and feel yourself stopping to struggle. In other words, *feel* acceptance. Take a deep breath in through your nose and let it out slowly through your mouth. Go to your own corner of the world and allow feelings of acceptance to flow through you. However anxious you may feel, relax and breathe through it. Remember, deep breathing alone can change your brain chemistry and increase calming neurotransmitters. Go ahead, take a deep breath and feel your body relax as you release it. If you did, you felt the birth of healing and recovery. Learning to accept, and not to fight, is the foundation for total recovery. Continued acceptance will lead you to peaceful serenity.

At first, be prepared for your healing to come slowly. You will have up and down days and that is part of acceptance. If you have a very stressful day, expect some physical symptoms, but they will pass. Healing your mind and body after a long illness or traumatic episode takes time, acceptance, and understanding. Do not let down days throw you off and cause you to become discouraged. In the early stages of healing, you may feel like you are in a falling elevator. Time, patience, acceptance, and understanding are your special keys that will open any door.

You have walked the path of suffering, both physically and emotionally, and now your life will change. You will know the true meaning of health, happiness, and peace of mind. Why you were chosen to take this long and painful journey you may never know, but then again maybe you will if a loved one reaches out for help. The path is never as dark or lonely when someone who cares reaches out to you.

At first, your healing comes gradually in waves. You may feel gloriously peaceful one day and in turmoil the next. In the peaceful moments you may think, "I'm healed." If a stressful event occurs, your nerves at this stage continue to register stress too intensely. It takes time for sensitization to heal. Understand this and never be discouraged by slow recovery in the early stages. Time and acceptance are always the answers. You now have a key to understanding.

Suffering like yours, in many ways, is a special experience. You learn by contrast. Until you have known emotional pain, you never know the true meaning of peace, and God knows, you know pain.

Post traumatic stress and chronic emotional fatigue attack those who cannot express, sort out, or deal with stress, anxiety, depression, fear, or grief. Do not repress. Express. Declare yourself to those who are trying to take control of your life. I have found health, happiness, and peace of mind are the keys to the best quality of life you could ever dream of. Peace be with you. *Let your healing begin.*

Emotional Trauma

Emotional trauma occurs when a traumatic experience leaves indelible memories in the brain to which a person continually returns. The memories, nightmares, fears, and flashbacks all remain the hallmark symptoms of emotional trauma. Individuals who have experienced emotional trauma will go to great lengths to avoid places, people, or any activity that reminds them of the traumatic event.

During the first four to six weeks after the event, the symptoms will be diagnosed as acute stress disorder and a treatment program will be given that addresses the symptoms. Most people respond to specific amino acids and behavior therapy for emotional trauma. Flashbacks will occur if a particular stimulus sets off the amygdala in the brain's limbic system. Dreams, noises, smells, similar tragic events, or any new trauma can trigger old unresolved trauma. If symptoms persist beyond six weeks, the diagnosis then becomes post traumatic stress disorder.

Many doctors feel the time since the event is the determining factor, but my research supports the emotional state of the person. If you are experiencing illness or any type of stressful event, you are more prone to post traumatic stress disorder long-term. This could most certainly cause the start of chronic emotional fatigue. When a traumatic event occurs, the sympathetic nervous system is activated and memories are tagged or encoded. Those who experience post traumatic stress disorder develop a short circuit in the information processing system. When incoming information is deemed unsafe or fearful, the short circuit causes repeated and intense stimulation of the *fight-or-flight* system. Behavior studies have shown that the logical part of the cortex shuts down when a person becomes hyper aroused leaving them feeling very vulnerable, fearful, anxious, and almost out of control. Post traumatic stress disorder sufferers have very high serum cortisol levels that cause anxiety and panic attacks. Cortisol causes the heart to beat faster and in many cases hyperventilation follows.

If you have experienced a traumatic episode and feel you cannot get a handle on it, then it is time to a find sympathetic therapist to help you, but find one that does not use psychiatric drugs. The amino acids and nutrient protocol I have used on hundreds of patients are very effective. Drugs only block symptoms and cause you to live a passive existence. You need to be very active in your healing and feel as though you have climbed the mountain, not stay below and wonder if you will ever feel good again.

Symptoms of F
ar
Chronic Emotiona.

1. Anxiety
2. Mood swings
3. Mental and physical fatigue
4. Sluggishness
5. Chronic muscle spasms
6. Uncertainty
7. Fear that comes and goes
8. Panic attacks
9. Sleep problems
10. Chronic digestive upset
11. Constant body aches and pains
12. Stiff neck and / or limited range of motion
13. Muscle jerks
14. Churning stomach
15. Eye strain
16. Loss of interest
17. No sex drive
18. Pounding heart, skipped beats
19. Low self esteem
20. No conn.
21. Withdrawal
22. Sensitivity to bright lights
23. Sensitivity to noise, especially loud sounds
24. Depression
25. Tension headaches or other headaches.
26. Constant stress
27. Blurred vision
28. Constant fear of failure
29. Feelings of helplessness and hopelessness
30. Feelings of guilt
31. As fatigued in the morning upon awakening as when you went to bed.
32. Apathy
33. Tension

tress and Post Trauma Levels

Stress is a subjective and personal effect. What is stressful to you may not be to someone else. People react differently to various situations. Just because something does not cause stress to others does not mean it might not be stressful to you. Stress triggers can come from a variety of sources including overwork, addiction in either yourself or a loved one, death of a loved one, divorce, lack of sleep, changes or loss of employment, increased use of tranquilizers, antidepressants or pain medications, unexpected illness or anything that taxes you mentally or physically. Both positive and negative stressors are taxing, even if a change is for the good. It may involve readjustments, uncertainty and anxiety. Other sources of stress might be negative thinking habits, a high-strung or impulsive character, emotional drains, social pressures, conflicts, confusion, frustration, loneliness and boredom. Even certain diseases, injuries, pain, chemical or radiation exposure, and drugs can be the catalyst for stress. The warning signal for danger comes when small stresses begin to combine, multiplying their effects, especially when they remain unresolved.

The Symptoms of Stress

Over the past ten years we have done extensive research at the Pain & Stress Center on the physical and mental effects of stress. Stress causes a slow deterioration of your immune system and your mental functioning. One day you just cannot seem to get it all together, and you are overwhelmed by fear and confusion that add to the effects of stress.

The first level of symptoms is very slight. Symptoms can be as mild as losing interest in doing enjoyable activities, consuming too much alcohol, sagging of the corners of the eyes. Additional symptoms include becoming short-tempered, boredom, nervousness, rolling of your hands, or developing creases in your forehead. These are evidence that the brain and body are dealing with more than they can handle. At this point you should stop and evaluate your lifestyle and see what changes you can make. Take control of your life.

The second level of symptoms is more noticeable. They include tiredness, angry outbursts, insomnia, loss of interest, fears, sadness, nagging anxiety, loss of sex drive, changes in eating habits, and withdrawal. These important warning signs indicate you are not handling your stress. Changes should be made immediately to reverse the cycle. Evaluate your lifestyle, diet and nutrients. If you cannot make the necessary changes, seek a therapist to help you.

The third level of symptoms includes physical symptoms: aches all over, muscle spasms, headaches, neck and back pain, high blood pressure, crying, digestive problems, strange heartbeats, facial tics, never feeling well, constant anxiety and depression, inability to concentrate, use of antidepressants, pain medications, tranquilizers, or daily alcohol ingestion. These signs are evidence that the stress is having a serious effect on your body and mind. Immediate actions should be taken to make changes; get professional assistance.

The fourth level of symptoms can result in actual disease

such as heart disease, cancer, skin disorders, ulcers, asthma, stroke, hepatitis, kidney failure, chronic allergies, susceptibility to infection, chronic pain, or mental breakdown. All of these have, in many cases, been related to prolonged stress.

Many times some diseases can be reversed by eliminating the stress, taking needed nutrients and amino acids, or getting the right therapy. Sometimes they can be brought on by other factors but greatly aggravated by additional stress conditions. Often, even the condition itself creates additional stress, and therefore aggravates the condition.

Disease is now coming to be seen as arising from causes within the person such as nutrient imbalances and the body's reaction to environmental changes. People have begun to take direct responsibility for their health. Our interest in nutrition is a symbol of this health change of attitude. The functions of amino acids are the most diverse of any of the nutrient groups. They contribute to the formation of proteins, muscles, and neurotransmitters that are the chemical language of the brain. Stress demands more amino acids because they are burned so rapidly.

The Adrenal Fatigue Factor

Adrenal fatigue affects up to 80% of the population at some point in their lifetime. Adrenal fatigue is the primary cause of burn out and stressed out, brain fatigue. Most physicians listen to all of the symptoms presented by patients then diagnose their problem as chronic fatigue. The adrenal glands located on top of each kidney, in the back, are about the size of a walnut and weigh less than a grape. The adrenals are the stress-response organs that help your body respond to stress so you can cope and survive. The adrenals are small pod shaped organs that are the major steroid factories of the body. They produce numerous vital hormones essential to health and energy production. The adrenals secrete exact amounts of steroid hormones that help minimize negative influences such as chronic stress, alcohol and environmental allergens. If chronic stress, trauma, or depression continues, the adrenals release too much cortisol into the bloodstream; this causes your brain and body to overcompensate and more problems can occur.

According to William Regelson, M.D. in his book, *The Super Hormone Promise,* the adrenals are the major producer of DHEA or Dehydroepiandrosterone. Dr. Regelson reports that DHEA rejuvenates the immune system, improves brain function and relieves stress. DHEA treats menopausal symptoms, restores memory, and enhances libido. DHEA is the super hormone of the 21st century.

DHEA levels drop steadily as we age suggesting that DHEA may be a biomarker or measure of the aging process. Dr. Regelson goes on to explain that DHEA sulfate levels change as we age. We peak in our twenties and the level

DHEA Sulfate Levels and Aging

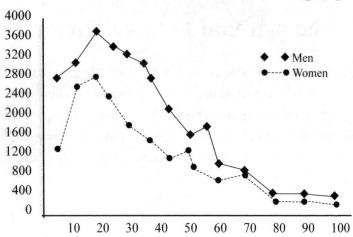

declines by half at age 40. The level continues to drop every year. The best way to know exactly what you need is to have a DHEA sulfate level run. Ask your doctor to order the test; it is just a simple blood draw that explains exactly what you have and how much you need to take daily.

Dr. Jim Wilson, author of *Adrenal Fatigue: The 21st Century,* reports adrenal fatigue affects a major portion of the adult population during their natural life. According to Dr. Wilson, the hormones secreted by the adrenals influence all major processes in your body. They closely affect how carbohydrates and fats are converted into energy, the distribution of stored fat, and regulation of blood sugar. Dr. Wilson explains adrenal fatigue occurs when the adrenals are too stressed out to respond to daily stress. He outlines a list of common symptoms of adrenal fatigue such as chronic fatigue, decreased immune response, fear, anxiety, depression, arthritis pain, insomnia, memory loss, menopausal problems, P.M.S., and hypoglycemia.

Having personally tried DHEA I can tell you first hand, it

makes a world of difference in how I feel and how I handle patients all day as well as do research and write. I usually check my DHEA level twice a year so I can make adjustments, if needed. Using DHEA and Pregnenolone are my natural answer to hormone replacement therapy.

Pregnenolone is also a super hormone that can be taken with DHEA. Pregnenolone is the ultimate parent steroid precursor. The body produces all the steroid hormones from pregnenolone. A precursor means that pregnenolone allows your body decide how much DHEA and other hormones it requires.

Some scientists believe pregnenolone is a very potent

Pregnenolone and DHEA Pathways

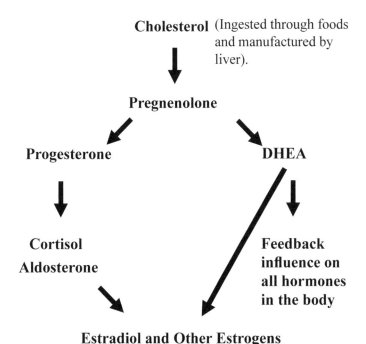

Cholesterol (Ingested through foods and manufactured by liver).

Pregnenolone

Progesterone

DHEA

Cortisol
Aldosterone

Feedback influence on all hormones in the body

Estradiol and Other Estrogens
Testosterone

Source: *DHEA, The Youth and Health Hormone* by C. Norman Shealy, M.D., p 4.

Hormone Deficiency Symptoms

DHEA Deficiency

Chronic fatigue, low bone density, difficulty losing weight, mood swings, sparse hair, illness, depressed immune system, any major disease, heart disease.

DHEA Excess

Acne or oily skin, increased facial hair, deepening of the voice, mood swings.

Hydrocortisone Deficiency

Fatigue, weakness, nausea, anorexia, hypotension, low blood sugar.

Hydrocortisone Excess

Obesity, thinning or bruising skin, slow wound healing, hypertension, osteoporosis, anxiety, sleep disorders.

Progesterone Deficiency

Headaches, low libido, anxiety, swollen breasts, moodiness, fuzzy thinking, depression, irritability, insomnia, cramps, emotional swings, inability to concentrate, painful joints, painful breasts, bloating, weight gain.

Progesterone Excess

Drowsiness, menstrual cycle changes.

Testosterone Deficiency

Depression, low or absent libido, lethargy, weakness, foggy thinking.

Testosterone Excess

Acne, fluid retention, weight gain, male hair growth patterns, exaggerated mood, aggression, impatience, frustration.

Source: "The Role of Hormone Testing" *Women's Health Connection.* Vol. 9 No. 1, p.2.

memory enhancer. Pregnenolone synthesizes from cholesterol. Cholesterol is a critical component for the production of steroid hormones. Both the brain and adrenal cortex produce pregnenolone. As with DHEA, pregnenolone also declines with age. As your pregnenolone production drops so does our production of other vital hormones.

Many scientists suggest that pregnenolone's effect on mental function may be cumulative. Super hormones are similar to neurotransmitters and have a very positive effect on brain function. Pregnenolone enhances the effects of GABA and restores a balance to your brain. One question I am asked constantly, "How long does it take to feel the effects of DHEA and pregnenolone?" That answer depends on how low your level is and how stressed your adrenals are; usually in 10 days to 2 weeks, you begin to pick up and feel more like taking part in familiar activities. DHEA and pregnenolone are not magic bullets, but they help you restore your brain and body with the nutrients you need to maintain healthy adrenal glands.

Special Note: If you have had a post traumatic experience in the last year and your energy level is low, have your DHEA sulfate level checked as soon as possible. Trauma can wipe out your adrenal function and keep you from healing. Begin taking 100 mg of Coenzyme Q10 every morning as soon as possible. The CoQ10 supports your heart and increases your energy. Increase your serotonin by taking 5-HTP on a daily basis, preferably at bedtime. You can use a full dropper of Liquid Serotonin throughout the day as needed. Remember, serotonin is the master controller in the brain, and it cannot be stored. It must be taken on a daily basis to maintain the needed level your brain requires. For small adults less than 100 pounds or children, use HTP10 to elevate your serotonin level; if you weigh over 100 pounds, use Mood Sync.

Your Hungry Brain

Everything that happens in your brain—every thought, every memory, even the will to move a muscle happens because of the release of neurotransmitters. Neurotransmitters come from amino acids, the chemical language of the brain. If you have low levels of neurotransmitters, your brain activity reflects it in your speech, memory, moods, and behavior. Your body uses amino acids and enzymes to breakdown foods into basic nutrients that are absorbed by billions of villi in your small intestine. If you take all the water and fat out of the body, amino acids make up 75% of what is left. Everything from the neurochemicals that are responsible for brain function to the protein your body uses to run and rebuild itself are created from amino acids.

Your hungry brain depends on your body's overall nutritional status for effective performance. Brain neurons consume 5 times more glucose than other cells. The neurons are busy every second of every day. The brain must have a healthy balance of nutrients to produce the energy it needs.

If you feel brain drain, look back at your diet. If it consists of junk food, your brain function reflects it. The brain must depend on the GI tract to assimilate and deliver needed nutrients that act as essential building blocks for neurotransmitters. Amino acids should be taken on a daily basis to keep the supply to the brain at optimum level.

You are what you eat, and your brain function depends on what you absorb. A balanced neurotransmitter complex gives your brain a boost, especially if your diet is unbalanced, or you have taken a lot of medication. Today, we know that our behavior and moods, both normal and disturbed, are the result of neurotransmitter processes going on within the brain. Alter the neurotransmitters, and your behavior and moods will be altered.

Serotonin is the master controller in the brain. Serotonin synthesizes from the amino acid, 5-HTP. 5-HTP derives from Griffonia seed, a natural plant source.

Tryptophan → 5-HTP → Serotonin, Master Controller

5-HTP is about 10 times stronger than tryptophan, and it is one step closer to serotonin. Neurotransmitters are the chemical substances that convey impulses from one neuron to another cell such as a muscle cell. Your hungry brain is made up of billions of neurons. Neurons are very specialized in their specific function; they allow your brain to learn, reason, and remember. Because of the activity of the neurons, the body responds and adjusts to changes in your environment. The stimuli respond with impulses that are directed at our sense organs: the eyes, ears, taste, and smell. The sensory receptors are located in the skin, muscles, bones, joints, and other parts of the body. Neurons or nerve cells are the brains of the nervous system that get fuel from neurotransmitters, serotonin, norepinephrine, acetylcholine, glutamine, and GABA. How you feed your hungry brain is evident everyday in how you think, feel, and are able to handle life's stresses and strains.

Traumatic Stress Headaches and Chronic Pain

Traumatic headaches and pain cannot be ascribed to a single mechanism but rather numerous encoded memories and experiences that activate chemical messages from the amygdala. Emotional trauma profoundly affects the information processing system. This short circuit effect causes a person to stay in a *fight-or-flight* cycle.

At the Pain & Stress Clinic to reduce muscle tension headaches, and pain, we use several modalities. They include ice/heat, behavior and orthomolecular therapies, biofeedback/relaxation, IV magnesium when needed, massage, manipulation, magnetic therapy, and TENS (Transcutaneous Electrical Nerve Stimulation) units. The overall response is good. The treatment modalities run 6 to 24 weeks. The orthomolecular therapy is continued on an ongoing basis and is designed to meet individual's needs. The overall success with the patients in the program is 85%.

Post traumatic headaches and pain occur as a result of micro traumas or any injury such as an accident, fall, or other activities. An injury from an accident, such as a whiplash, occurs when a person is hit in such a way that it causes a hyperextension or hyperflexion of the head and neck. Whiplash causes tremendous stress and strain on the supporting muscles, ligaments, and bones. In these cases, implement pain therapy as well as nutritional therapy and psychotherapy is used. Relaxation training is excellent because it teaches you to relax

Traumatic Stress Headaches and Chronic Pain Physical Symptoms

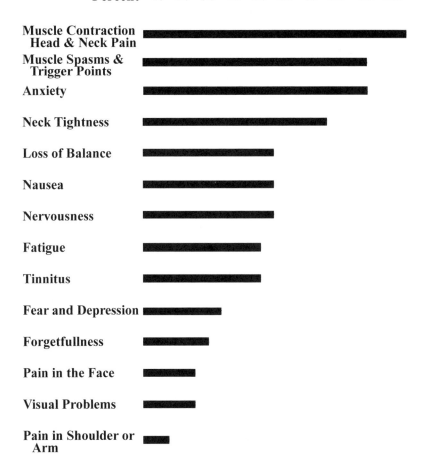

During in-depth evaluations 250 patients described these physical symptoms. Ages varied from 25 to 65 with 75% of the patients being women and 25% men. All experienced some type of trauma prior to the onset of symptoms.

tight muscles in spasm and how to relax rather than become tense, especially when first starting to drive after an accident. The tendency is to become tense and hyper vigilant causing muscles to contract and spasm.

Tension headaches caused by stress and trauma affect up to 20% of the population and occur in this population at least once a week. The most common cause of tension headaches is the prolonged and sustained contraction of the shoulder, neck, and head muscles. The pain usually refers up from the shoulder muscles into the neck muscles and forms what is commonly known as a trigger point. The more frequently the muscles are held in a contracted state combined with stress and trauma, the more the pain cycle repeats itself. Tension or muscle contraction headaches begin from a drop in brain chemicals such as serotonin, GABA, glutamine, and magnesium. Two critical neurotransmitters involved in the perception of pain are serotonin and endorphins. Serotonin regulates the diameter of the blood vessels and anxiety/stress reactions. Endorphins are the brain's natural morphine as well as dopamine and acetylcholine that balance the brain chemistry.

The tendency of most headache sufferers is to reach for a heating pad, but this does not decrease pain and swelling as ice does. Use an ice pack for 20 minutes on an area, remove for 30 minutes, then reapply, if needed. Go to the source of the pain such as the shoulder or neck muscles that are referring

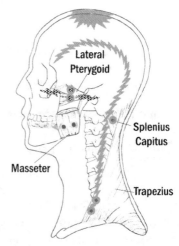

Headache Trigger Points

pain to the head. Do not hesitate to use massage along with osteopathic or chiropractic manipulation for relief.

Analyze what is causing your headaches and obtain the necessary professional treatment you need. I do not encourage self-diagnosis. You need an objective evaluation and a progressive treatment plan to help restore your injured and traumatized body in the healing process. This may include modifications in your life that have a negative effect on your brain and body. Many times you are unaware that a particular activity can be the cause of chronic pain. This is why I encourage a professional evaluation. In summary, your answer for tension headaches, chronic neck, shoulder, or back pain lies in a combination approach utilizing all of the various modalities.

From personal experience I can tell you continuing pain therapy makes a major difference in your life. After 25 years of collegiate and professional tennis, as well as other sports, my body really needed all the help it could get. Then to top it off, I was hit from behind on the expressway by a gravel truck, so now I have the trauma and the injury. Today, I am able to function and do all of the many things my busy life calls for because I get regular chiropractic manipulation, massage, and take amino acids and nutrients on a daily basis. And I never ever forget my magnesium. When I asked my chiropractor about the reoccurring shoulder pain, as well as other little problems, especially after 50, he said, "It's the sins of the past and the demands of the present." His observation is right on the money.

Post Traumatic Stress and Chronic Emotional Fatigue And The Immune System

In the last several decades scientists have turned their attention to the immune system as the major foundation of health. The immune system is the ultimate basis of how you feel and how your mind and body are able to handle your stress, chemical pollution, prescription drugs, and poor nutrition. Infections call the immune system into action. The ingenious design of the immune system ensures the ready availability and quick assembly of an immune response anywhere it is needed. The immune system works throughout the entire body to fight bacterial, viral, and fungal (yeast) infections responsible for illnesses such as the common cold and the flu.

When you have an infection the body must fight it off, so the immune system sounds the alarm and sends repeated messages to the brain to activate and increase in number the body's white blood cells. White blood cells are the major cells of the immune system that ingest microbes, antigens, and other substances. An antigen is any substance that stimulates an immune system response. Chronic stress, fatigue, anxiety, depression, and grief weaken your immune system. Your state of mind and positive thinking increase the overall state of your immune system. Remember, whatever the brain tells the body to do, it does.

The brain's stress response system is activated in times of crisis. Your immune system responds automatically to pathogens and foreign molecules that try to invade the body. The major response symptoms are the body's special means for maintaining an internal ultimate state of homeostasis—the process of maintaining physiological and psychological balance in the body.

Tissues and cells involved with immune function are highly energy dependent and therefore require an adequate supply of Coenzyme Q10 for optimal function. There are numerous clinical studies that document the immune enhancing effect of CoQ10. Immune function tends to decline with age and illness. Thus, CoQ10 and other nutrient supplementation help prevent or even reverse age-related immunosuppression.

In clinical studies patients with chronic fatigue, stress exhaustion, post surgical fatigue, and trauma showed a remarkable improvement using 300 mg of CoQ10 daily for 120 days. CoQ10 supplementation can reverse the deficiency state and helps prevent toxicity to the heart muscle. Standard doses taken on a daily basis should be at least 150 mg daily. According to Stephen Sinatra, M.D., author of *The Coenzyme Q10 Phenomenon,* "Aging is a complex biological process involving a progressive decline in the biochemical performance of specific tissues and organs, the potential for Coenzyme Q10 as an antioxidant, membrane-stabilizer and support for ATP synthesis may slow down the physiological and biological decline that occurs with aging."

Other important antioxidants are Vitamin E. Investigators found 27% of adults have low blood concentrations of Vitamin E, increasing their risk for developing cardiovascular disease and cancer. In the August 1999 *American Journal of Epidemiology,* a report focused on a study of 16,295 U.S. adults, aged 18 and over. African Americans had the lowest Vitamin E levels. The same journal reported a connection between low E levels and memory loss. Adults older than 60 found that decreasing serum levels were consistently associated with increasing levels of poor memory.

For my patients I use the following on a daily basis to

support the immune system.

1. **CoQ10,** 150 mg in the morning with food.
2. **Vitamin E**, 400 I.U. in the morning.
3. **Deluxe Scavengers,** 1 in the morning, and 2 in the evening.
4. **NAC 600** mg, 1 capsule, twice daily.
5. **Alpha Lipoic Acid 300 mg,** 1 capsule, twice daily.
6. **Olive Leaf Extract 500 mg,** 1 every 8 hours. Use D-Lenolate Olive Leaf Extract, as it is the patented, studied form and twice as potent as other olive leaf extracts. It is best that you only use Olive Leaf for 10 days to 2 weeks.
7. **Ester C 500 mg with Bioflavonoids** capsules, 6 capsules, twice daily.
8. **Beta Glucan 75 mg,** 2 capsules twice to three times daily for 2 weeks.

Why We Will Never Forget 9-11!

9-11 changed the lives of every man, woman, and child in this country, and even if you live to be 100, you will never forget it. Why? As you watched in disbelief the events unfold, your brain and body recorded every minute detail. As you watched on television, the sight and sounds were the major brain imprint. If you live the New York area, not only the sight and sound were imprinted in the brain, but the smell and touch as well. According to Candace Pert, Ph.D., author of *Molecules of Emotion*, intelligence and memory are in every cell of your body. The mind is not confined to the brain; the mind is throughout the brain and body. Dr. Pert's research demonstrates the chemicals that run our body and brains are the same chemicals that are involved in emotion. The mind and body are one; they are inseparable. The anger, depression, and grief you felt on 9-11 was felt in every cell of your body and recorded. When events from 9-11 or any traumatic event play back, the symptoms can affect any part of your body. This is how past trauma works. Short-or-long term traumatic emotions affect our immune system as well as our mental state. When a full-blown flashback occurs, the amygdala begins sending signals, and the body responds with a full-blown *fight-or-flight* response. The adrenal glands on the kidneys begin pumping adrenaline that trigger fear reactions all over the body. A sudden rush of adrenaline and noradrenaline (norepinephrine) cause your heart to pound, your breathing becomes shallow, pupils widen and dilate, and your mouth feels like it is full of cotton. If you have had other traumatic events, your amygdala is on overload and your neurotransmitters are deficient. Your symptoms will be worse with nausea, feelings of diarrhea, dizziness, profuse sweating, trembling, and hyperventilation. At this point you get a lactate buildup in your muscles, and your arms feel like they have lead in them.

There was nothing normal about the events that unfolded on 9-11. There was nothing to compare it to. You experience an abnormal reaction to an abnormal situation that is repeated over and over, for years to come. You will dwell on the events, and your fear as well as your uncertainty will intensify. What you experienced is locked in every cell of your body, and the physical effects bring forth new pain from past trauma.

Does post trauma stress cause chronic emotional fatigue? Post trauma is locked into the cells of your brain and body. Traumatic events can playback at any time, especially if events stimulate the specific areas of the brain where long-term memories are stored. Research demonstrates that teens and younger children at the time of a particular trauma have a strong possibility of re-experiencing the trauma, especially if it was prolonged.

An example of this is the Columbine High School shooting in Colorado. Many teens and parents still have nightmares and flashbacks. All of their senses were affected; they had nothing to compare it to, nor anyway to rationalize it. What happened to them in this state of mind can be recalled in the same state of mind. This means anytime you are in an extreme stressful or anxious state of mind, your amygdala can begin playing old tapes or releasing messages from previous traumas. When you witness the traumatic death of a friend or loved one, your brain and body reach down to their deepest core. Within that deep core of the limbic system, the amygdala stores that experience in every cell of your brain and body.

Research studies from UCLA demonstrate if all the impressions and memories of the brain of a 50-year-old person could be recorded on tape, the length of the tape would reach to the moon and back several times. When you stop and think of how much information is stored in your brain, you begin to understand how it affects your physical being.

The mind is a powerful tool, but it can also be a powerful weapon.

The Healing Process

Understanding what is going on inside of you is one of the most important steps you will take in healing. Being real and enjoying listening to yourself to accept who you are with no regrets is closing wounds. Most people carry too much of the past with them and internalize low esteem messages, negativity which comes from parents, teachers, peers, and even loved ones. Healing means you don't block a thought or situation, whether it is pleasant or not. You come to terms with it. You deal with it. It means understanding and being comfortable with how you feel. It means being in touch with for the first time in your life those feeling that you have held inside. If you can be real in relationships with friends and family and express your true feelings, you will advance the depth of the relationship because the truth that you give them is what they have been looking for in themselves.

You will feel a deep sense of satisfaction when you communicate your true self to someone you love. This might not be easy at first because you experience changes from day to day. It will take some adjustments to be able to communicate your pain from the past. Releasing the pain of the past is tied into the act of forgiveness. You may not feel it in those terms, but those terms are the ones that allow you to feel free and live your life to its fullest. You are the only one who can free yourself from the pain of the past.

True forgiveness is letting go of hurt. The healing process involves your ability to forgive someone by telling him or her the pain they caused you no longer hurts. The importance is not the event or the person who hurt you but how you choose to react to it. True healing from the pain of unexpressed feelings and anger of the past is your expression of those feelings without hesitation in the present so that the present has the power to help heal you. Expressing what is real that lives inside of you will allow you to feel genuine, spontaneous, and more alive than you ever felt before. Everyone is guilty to some extent of allowing fear to control what they say, so they repress, hold it in, and become a victim of their own fear and their painful past. Does this begin the cycle of chronic emotional fatigue and a possible disease state? Yes! Your life should not be a passive process in which you depend on others but rather an active process generated from within. Living in the past is existence. You need to be in a place of acceptance. What has happened, has happened—it is only happening now because you allow it to. Cross the time line to the past and let the pain of the past, stay in the past. Your healing process has begun!

Amino Acids for Brain and Body Function

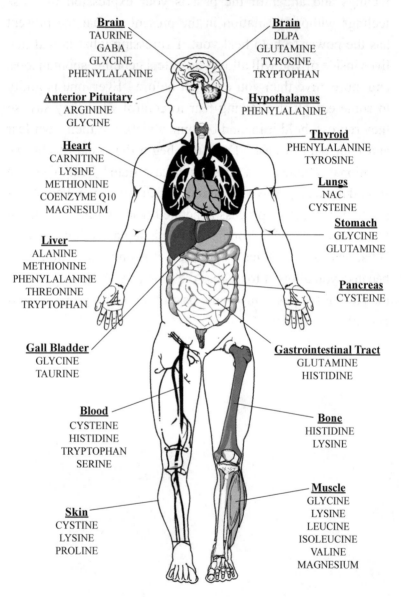

Brain
TAURINE
GABA
GLYCINE
PHENYLALANINE

Brain
DLPA
GLUTAMINE
TYROSINE
TRYPTOPHAN

Anterior Pituitary
ARGININE
GLYCINE

Hypothalamus
PHENYLALANINE

Thyroid
PHENYLALANINE
TYROSINE

Heart
CARNITINE
LYSINE
METHIONINE
COENZYME Q10
MAGNESIUM

Lungs
NAC
CYSTEINE

Stomach
GLYCINE
GLUTAMINE

Liver
ALANINE
METHIONINE
PHENYLALANINE
THREONINE
TRYPTOPHAN

Pancreas
CYSTEINE

Gall Bladder
GLYCINE
TAURINE

Gastrointestinal Tract
GLUTAMINE
HISTIDINE

Blood
CYSTEINE
HISTIDINE
TRYPTOPHAN
SERINE

Bone
HISTIDINE
LYSINE

Skin
CYSTINE
LYSINE
PROLINE

Muscle
GLYCINE
LYSINE
LEUCINE
ISOLEUCINE
VALINE
MAGNESIUM

Always add magnesium and B6 or P5'P to all amino acids.

Stress Reduction Exercise

Read this stress reduction exercise as often as possible to train yourself to breath through stressful events.

Direct your attention to your breathing.

Not the thought of the breathing but the direct sensation of the breathing as the air enters and leaves by itself.

Let the awareness come right to the edge of sensation as the breath enters and leaves the nostrils.

Let the awareness be soft and open, making contact with each breath without the least interference.

Experience the natural tides of the breath, as it comes and goes. Do not attempt to change or control it. Just observe it.

Open to receive each changing sensation that accompanies the breath, moment to moment.

Let the breath breathe itself, without comment or without any attempt to control it in anyway. Allow the breath to be as it is. If it is slow, let it be slow. If it is deep, let it be deep. If it is shallow, let it be shallow. Allow awareness and sensation to meet, moment to moment, with each inhalation and with each exhalation.

Let the breath be completely natural and free, in no way held by the mind. Just let the breath breathe itself. Sensations arise, instant to instant, in the vast spaciousness of awareness.

If you notice the mind attempting to shape the breath, to control it in even the least way, just watch that tendency and let the breath float free. No holding. No control.

Completely let go of the breath. Let the body breath by itself. Do not interfere with the subtle flow, just awareness as vast as the spacious sky.

The sensations of the breath arise and pass away within this openness . . . nothing to hold to . . . nothing to do . . . just the breath as it is.

Float, drift, relax, and return to this peaceful state as often as you want.

When you repress or suppress

those things which you

don't want to live with ...

you don't really solve the problem

because you don't bury

the problem dead,

you bury it alive!

It remains alive and

active inside of you.

Negative Thinking Yields Chronic Stress and Emotional Fatigue

1. When you feel you have a *negative* mood, it means you are feeling down or depressed. It causes a sense of pessimism and unhappiness.
2. Some *negative* moods are normal and cannot be avoided totally. Do not dwell on this. Work through it as soon as possible.
3. *Negative* moods as with any mood can be changed. They are not permanent, even though you feel like it will last forever.
4. Many *negative* moods are the result of illogical, irrational, and uncertainty in thinking. For example, you will never get better and be free of anxiety.
5. Change *Negative* moods by focusing on what you want to do, not what you are experiencing now.
6. Focusing on and thinking about *negative* feelings does not change the feelings. You are playing old tapes from your past.
7. Change how you think (self-talk) and what you do (your behavior) will change your feelings and give you better control of your life.
8. If you start to think negatively, stop and reverse the behavior pattern. Go to your own corner of the world and relax. Get in touch with the negativity and why you are thinking negatively.
9. If you do not believe you can change your thoughts or behaviors, chances are your thoughts and behaviors will not change.
10. You are what you are and what you believe you can make happen. Whenever you feel negative feelings, let them go. Don't dwell! *Resolve it and let it go!*

The Art of Feeling Good
and Letting Go

If your moods and emotions are continuously clouded by the experiences of the past, you have not let go of the past. You must be free in the present to enjoy the present. Release the past, and let it rest in peace. Stay in the present where you have control.

When a negative mood occurs, identify what your thoughts are at the time. Does it follow a stressful day? Did you get angry? Did you feel out of control? Don't worry. Just accept it and let it go. You are the master of your thoughts.

Take time to reflect and acknowledge the positive things that occur in your life. When you feel down, you tend to forget the positive events that have happened. Allow your mental filter to sort thoughts and drain the negative or traumatic thoughts.

If you feel fatigue and negative feelings when you think of experiences and relationships in the past, it's because letting go of the past and the pain that comes with it is tied into the act of forgiveness. Maybe you are not aware of this emotional link, but it is something you must consider and act on if you want peace and healing.

How you handle negative criticism or a threat of negative criticism in your adult life correlates with the ego strength you developed in the interactions with your very first and most important critics.

As a child you begin to store all the negative inputs; this is because you hear more don't than dos, and you hear more fear than strength. For many who spend their childhood holding off a steady stream of negative criticism, the damage has been done. You do not erase that old tape. You continue to play it back, the fear of failure grows stronger, and the chronic stress continues and fatigue takes over.

Your goal must be to direct total control over your life and the ability to let go of negative feelings, hurt, and pain. Live each day to it's fullest.

Journey Through PTSD

The weather was bad, so I decided to take the bus home rather than drive and fight the weather and heavy traffic. About ten minutes out of town it happened—a big truck driving too fast lost control and hit us broadside. I don't remember anything until I woke up in the hospital. Every time I moved, the pain was so intense I wanted to scream, cry, and laugh all at the same time. The safety I sought on the bus left me wondering if there was any such thing as a *safe* journey. I drifted back into sleep trying to escape the pain and the fear that my broken body would never heal.

Six weeks later I was released from the hospital in a wheelchair. I was told I would have a long road ahead of me for all my broken bones and injuries to heal. The injury I wondered about, but no one would discuss, was my fear. The thoughts of driving, rain, and trucks left me in a panicked state. The doctors told me I should not drive for at least six months. I didn't know if I ever wanted to drive again.

When I opened the door to my home, everything was just as I had left it. My neighbor, a nurse, came over to cheer me up. She put a name on the feelings, fears, and anxiety that were consuming me—PTSD (Post Traumatic Stress Disorder)— prognosis and healing time unknown. I was lost in a sea of uncertainty that intensified my injuries. I was alive, but my brain was screaming, crying, and reaching out for help. The *tragedy* was that the only consolations doctors offered me were *drugs* (to make me forget) and the *advise*, *"Give it time, you'll be okay."*

PTSD was Star Wars in my head. I knew I had a long journey ahead of me, and I had to find the right help.

This is a brief profile of the hell PTSD sufferers live in. PTSD is a never-ending journey to heal the mind, so the body will follow.

Brain Distress Pathways

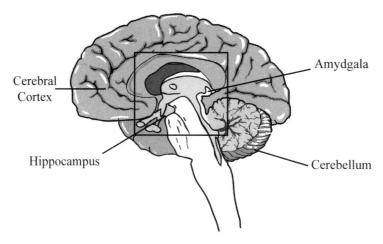

Cerebral Cortex

Amydgala

Hippocampus

Cerebellum

The limbic system is the region of the brain where emotion and moods are regulated and conveyed to the brain (cerebral cortex). The limbic system contains the inhibitory neurotransmitters, GABA, glutamine, glycine, and serotonin that modulate anxiety, fear, and pain messages in the brain. The limbic system functions as a crossover zone where signals are transmitted from the rest of the cortex into the limbic system. The complex and powerful amygdala, as part of the limbic system, is the storehouse of memories, emotions, and especially, traumatic experiences. Research documents the amygdala is functioning at birth; this accounts for negative experiences of our inner child that remain in the amygdala as unresolved anxiety, anger, and fear. The hippocampus plays a role in long-term memory, and is a storehouse of knowledge comparing the past and present while monitoring current events for coding into the brain.

Symptoms of Serotonin Deficiency

- Aggression
- Alcoholism
- Anxiety
- Carbohydrate cravings
- Chronic pain
- Depression
- Fibromyalgia
- Hyperactivity
- Insomnia
- Mood swings
- Migraine headaches
- Obesity
- Obsessive-compulsive disorder
- Panic attacks
- Violent behavior

Symptoms of Amino Acid Deficiencies

- ADD/ADHD
- Alcoholism
- Ammonia toxicity
- Ataxia (defective muscular coordination)
- Behavioral disorders
- Cardiovascular disease
- Chemical intolerances
- Chronic fatigue
- Chronic gastrointestinal distress or bowel irregularity
- Depression
- Dermatitis (inflammation of the skin)
- Detoxification impairments
- Excessive inflammation
- Failure to thrive (infancy)
- Family history or early symptoms of degenerative disease
- Frequent headaches
- Frequent infections and persistent inflammatory responses
- Hyperlipidemias (high blood lipid levels)
- Hypertension (high blood pressure)
- Hypotonia (loss of muscle tone)
- Inflammatory disorders
- Impaired mental development
- Insomnia
- Intolerances (persistent) to foods and chemicals
- Mental disperception
- Mental retardation
- Myopathies (muscular diseases)
- Neurological disorders
- Neural tube defects (birth defects)
- Ocular (eye) disorders
- Osteoporosis
- Oxidative stress
- Poor immunity
- Poor wound healing
- Rheumatoid arthritis
- Seizures
- Short stature or chronically underweight, growth failure (children)
- Weak skin and nails

Source: *Diagnostic Value of Amino Acid Analysis*, Great Smokies Diagnostic Laboratory, 2000

Nutritional Support Program For Post Trauma and Chronic Emotional Fatigue

Your diet should be one of your first considerations. It should be low in fat and simple carbohydrates, moderate in protein intake, and high in fiber. Many hidden substances usually high in fat and sugar are present in many processed foods. Become an informed consumer and a label reader.

The "cave man" diet is generally a good diet because it is high in fruits and vegetables, low in fat, and moderate in proteins. The foods are generally eaten without a great deal of preparation and in a more *whole* form. As an example, a baked potato is preferred over mashed or fried potatoes. The baked potato is higher in fiber and is high in complex carbohydrates. Simple carbohydrates such as sugar should be avoided. Simple carbohydrates raise your blood sugar rapidly giving you a false high. But this only lasts for a short time before your blood sugar plummets, and you hit bottom. If sugar is your downfall, try using some Gymnema Sylvestre, 1 capsule three times daily; if you are over 200 pounds, use 2 capsules, three times daily.

Do not eat fried foods, as your body has to work much harder to overcome the free radicals created by these foods. Fried foods equal high fat content. Limit the amount of fat you ingest. Stay with chicken, turkey, or fish, while only occasionally eating beef.

Limit your intake of caffeine. Caffeine has been linked

to increased anxiety and nervousness. Do not forget that most regular sodas are high in sugar and contain caffeine. Instead, try some water or herbal teas for a change.

Limit your ingestion of alcohol. Alcohol tends to be high in sugar. Again, it may relax you, but it can also backfire causing depression and anxiety, and it is habit forming. It can also cause havoc with your sinuses and allergies and further zap your energy.

Avoid smoking or smoke. Even inhalation of second-hand smoke causes problems with your energy level and contributes to free radicals in your body. Avoid it like the plague!

Consider food allergies if you have either environmental or airborne allergies or if you have problems with your sinuses. Food allergies can be a source of many underlying problems such as fatigue and lack of energy.

Post trauma and chronic emotional fatigue deplete the brain of amino acids that are the precursors for inhibitory neurotransmitters. Neurotransmitters are the chemical language of the brain that transmit billions of messages between neurons. The brain contains six million nerve cells, fully half of the body's entire supply. Excitatory neurotransmitters activate virtually all neurons in the central nervous system including the brain. Inhibitory neurotransmitters including GABA, glutamine, glycine, taurine, tyrosine, and 5-HTP deactivate the neurons. I will focus on inhibitory neurotransmitters for calming and stress reduction. Amino acids must have B6, P'5P (Pyridoxal '5 Phosphate), and magnesium as vital cofactors.

The following is the supplementation program used at the Pain & Stress Center for patients with chronic emotional fatigue. All of the patients showed a marked improvement using this program. Review the products described in this section.

Select the supplements that *fit your symptoms.*

You *do not need* to take all of the products described below.

Good Multivitamin such as Total Vites or Brain Link on a daily basis.

Liquid Magnesium (Mag Chlor 85) is a concentrated liquid providing 85 mg of magnesium per cubic centimeter (cc). The most common symptoms of magnesium deficiency are chronic neck, back, and shoulder pains with recurrent muscle spasms. Muscles cannot relax without magnesium. If you have constant muscle spasms, migraines, depression, exhaustion, arrhythmias, twitches, or tremors, you are probably magnesium deficient. Other symptoms besides chronic pain that are often helped or relieved by magnesium are anxiety and pain, nervousness, cold white fingers, insomnia, hypertension, excessive perspiration, body odor, and irregular heartbeats. Use 10 to 25 drops, two to three times per day in juice.

Several years ago, I had the opportunity to listen to Sherry Rogers, M.D. Dr. Rogers has done extensive research on magnesium and magnesium deficiencies. Dr. Rogers reported excellent results with her patients that had described the above symptoms using magnesium therapy (Mag Link). The key to finding the exact dose of magnesium that your body requires is to take it up to bowel tolerance. By this, I mean loose stools. If you experience loose stools, then back your dose down by 1 tablet or 5 drops; you usually begin to feel better within 48 hours. If you weigh up to 125 pounds, take Mag Link, 4 tabs, spread throughout the day. If you weigh over 125 pounds, take

2 Mag Link, twice to three times daily. If you prefer liquid, use 10 to 25 drops in water or juice, twice to three times daily if less than 125 pounds; if over 125 pounds, use 10 to 25 drops, three to four times daily.

Mood Sync is an amino acid inhibitory neurotransmitter formula that offers an alternative to addictive prescriptive drugs. Mood Sync provides the proper amino acids to address and restore the brain chemical imbalance caused by depression, anger, aggression, stress and anxiety, mood swings, and PMS. Mood Sync contains 5-HTP, Tyrosine, GABA, Taurine, Glutamine, and B6. *Special Note: Do not take Mood Sync if you are taking a SSRI (Selective Serotoin Reuptake Inhibitory) or MAO antidepressant.*

HTP10 is an amino acid complex that is designed for small adults or children. If your child (age 10 and under) suffers from post trauma, HTP10 would be the product of choice along with the Brain Link. *Do not take HTP10 if you are taking a SSRI (Selective Serotoin Reuptake Inhibitor) or MAO antidepressant.*

Tyrosine helps restore the brain chemistry from stress exhaustion. Tyrosine enhances neurotransmitters and lifts the symptoms of depression. Phenylalanine breaks down to tyrosine in the liver. Tyrosine is converted to dopa, then epinephrine, and norepinephrine. Most antidepressants work by increasing or manipulating the amount of norepinephrine in the brain. Tyrosine does this naturally, whereas most drugs have side effects. A word of warning, *if you are taking antidepressants, you cannot just stop taking them and start taking tyrosine.* Tyrosine or phenylalanine *CANNOT be combined with tricyclic or MAO inhibitors antidepressants or if you have a history of a melonoma.* Check with your pharmacist or physician. Tyrosine is available in 500 and 850 mg capsules. Dosage depends on a person's weight. If you weigh up to 125 pounds, use 1 Tyrosine 500 mg in the morning and afternoon; if over 125 pounds, use 1, 850 mg Tyrosine in the morning and in the afternoon.

Anxiety Control is a patented formula that restores the brain depleted by stress and anxiety. Anxiety Control contains GABA, Glycine, Glutamine, Passion Flower, Primula Officinalis, magnesium, and B6. Anxiety Control's special combination of amino acids activates the neurotransmitters needed by the brain replenishing the brain chemistry to its natural state. GABA, Glycine, and Glutamine are inhibitory neurotransmitters in the brain that slow the transmission of anxiety signals from the limbic system to the cortex or the thinking part of the brain. Many tranquilizers such as Valium and Xanax merely attach to the GABA receptor sites. GABA fills them. Stress depletes your GABA supply causing increased symptoms of anxiety and panic. Take Anxiety Control, 2 capsules, three times daily, and 2 at bedtime, if needed.

Sleep Link is the ultimate sleep formula that contains melatonin, L-Theanine, 5-HTP, GABA, Passion Flower, Ashwagandha, and Glutamine. Take 1 or 2 Sleep Link, 30 minutes before bedtime for sleep. *Special Note: Do not take Sleep Link if you are taking a SSRI (Selective Serotoin Reuptake Inhibitor) or MAO antidepressant.*

Sleep Link helps you obtain the restful sleep your body and brain require for repairs and healing. Sleep disorders occur when several brain chemicals or neuro-nutrients become out of balance due to chronic stress, anxiety, or depression. Sleep Link helps restore inhibitory neurotransmitter levels so any sleep disturbance you have resolves. Melatonin combined with the 5-HTP helps balance the circadian rhythm and release the accumulated stresses of the day. The pineal gland through its production of melatonin serves as a critical link between the brain and the immune system. A number of studies show that melatonin elevates the activity of certain types of immune system cells that are important in fighting infections. According to *Longevity,* October 1990, melatonin is especially effective in restoring the defenses of a person whose immune system has been weakened by stress. L-Theanine creates alpha waves in the brain and sends a message for the body and brain to relax.

For a *super bedtime cocktail*, combine 2 Sleep Link with Mag Chlor 85. Use 15 to 25 drops of the Mag Chlor in water or juice.

L–T™ is a combination of L-Theanine, GABA, and Glutamine. L-Theanine is the *relaxation amino acid*™ that is found in green leaves. L–T creates a calming effect in the brain without drowsiness or dull feelings. Studies show L-Theanine boosts brain waves reducing muscle tension, stress, and anxiety. Another study published in the *Journal of Food Science and Technology* verifies that L–T has a major effect on the release of neurotransmitters such as dopamine and serotonin. Take 1 to 2 capsules of L–T, three to four times per day as needed, to a maximum of 8.

Liquid Serotonin is a 1X homeopathic formula. For acute anxiety or stress, use 10 to 15 drops under the tongue as needed for calming.

Mellow Mind is 500 mg of Ashwagandha with Ester C. Ashwagandha or Indian ginseng promotes a calm sense of well-being while reducing tension, aches, and pains. Ashwagandha has sedative properties quieting the CNS (Central Nervous System) but energizes and fights fatigue, stress, and aging. Ashwagandha supports the immune system and promotes deep, dreamless sleep. Ashwagandha even improves sexual performance capacity. Suggested dose is 1 capsule of Mellow Mind, twice to three times daily.

Coenzyme Q10 (CoQ10) is a natural nutrient essential to the life and health of every cell. You cannot fight off infections without CoQ10 which decreases with age. Research indicates CoQ10 plays a critical role in the production of energy in almost every cell in the body and plays a major role in the treatment and prevention of serious diseases. Take 50 to 100 mg of CoQ10 daily.

Alpha KG and citric acid are components of the Krebs cycle. The Krebs cycle is the chemical engine that generates energy for every cell and gives the body *a kick start.* Alpha KG is a special formula for chronic fatigue and stress. Use 1 Alpha KG, twice daily for increased stamina and energy.

Ester C is a special Vitamin C that has a neutral pH or the same pH as distilled water. It does not cause the side effects often associated with large amounts of ascorbic acid. Ester C forms a metabolite with the body, so if you took a dose now, twenty-four hours later some of the C would still be present in your body. Vitamin C is important for the repair of body tissues and helps fight infections. Take a total of 2000 to 5000 mg of Ester C per day in divided doses.

Beta Glucan is a potent antioxidant that powerfully activates and strengthens the immune system. Studies at Harvard, Baylor College of Medicine, and MIT document that Beta Glucan increases the body's immune system by triggering specific white blood cells called macrophages. Your macrophages circulate in the body consuming any foreign invaders they meet. Beta Glucan helps your body resist infection, inhibits tumor growth, and enhances the effectiveness of antibiotics and antiviral medications.

Brain Link Complex is a neurotransmitter complex of

amino acids, vitamins, and minerals. Brain Link provides nutrients that are necessary for production of inhibitory neurotransmitters that control mind, mood, memory, and behavior. Supplement with Brain Link according to your weight. If you weigh less than 120 pounds, use 2 scoops of Brain Link Complex, twice daily; if you weigh over 120 pounds, use 3 scoops, twice daily.

Huperzine A is derived from a purified compound of Chinese club moss. Studies confirm Huperzine enhances memory by increasing the production of acetylcholine. Increased levels of acetylcholine produce better memory, concentration, and focus. Supplement with 1 Huperzine, twice a day.

Chromium and Carnitine is a combination formula that is important for the blood's sugar utilization, insulin production, fat distribution, and energy production. Chromium is a trace mineral that is vital for blood sugar regulation that works with insulin. In addition, chromium and carnitine assist in fat metabolism and play a part in cholesterol and triglycerides (fat levels) in the body. Carnitine provides energy in chronic fatigue. Chromium helps to keep blood sugar at normal levels. The usual dose of the Carnitine-Chromium combination is 1 to 2 caps per day.

Lysine is an amino acid that is important for the production of antibodies, hormones, and enzymes. Lysine is necessary for growth and tissue repair and helps modulate herpes attacks. Your skin reflects your emotions and stress level. The suggested dosage of lysine is 1000 to 1500 mg per day, divided, increasing to 3000 mg per day, divided for skin problems or herpes breakouts.

Pain Control is a natural analgesic with an anti-inflammatory herbal combination consisting of DLPA,

Boswellia, Ashwagandha, GABA, and B6. DLPA (DL-Phenylalanine) is an amino acid that helps with pain and depression. DLPA works by extending the lifespan of the body's endorphins or natural pain-killing substances. DLPA is not habit forming and works with other nutrients to reduce pain. *A note of caution if you are taking MAO or tricyclic antidepressants or have a history of melanoma, do not use Pain Control capsules or DLPA.* Boswellia provides pain relief by reducing inflammation for stress or tension pain and joint stiffness. Ashwagandha and GABA reduce muscle tension, stress, and anxiety. Use as needed; the usual dosage of Pain Control Capsules are 1 to 2 capsules every 4 to 6 hours as needed to a maximum of 8 capsules daily.

Pain Control Cream is an advanced pain relief formula that gives quick, lasting relief for knotted or overworked muscles, stress-tension, aches and pains, or overuse of joints. Pain Control Cream contains bromelain, emu oil, boswellia, glucosamine sulfate, MSM, and pregnenolone. When you apply Pain Control Cream to the skin, it quickly penetrates the skin for fast relief.

Boswella Plus is an herbal plus Ester C formula. Boswellia (Frankincense) and Ester C offer anti-inflammatory and pain reducing properties. Boswellia has been used for pain and inflammation for thousands of years. Boswellia offers a safe and effective alternative to the NSAIDs (Non-steroidal Anti-Inflammatory Drugs) without the stomach and gastrointestinal (GI) side effects of medications. The usual dosage of Boswellia is a 300 mg capsule, twice per day with food.

Scavenger Antioxidant Formula is a combination of beta-carotene, Vitamin C, Bioflavonoids, Rutin, Vitamin E, selenium, cysteine, and B6 (P 5' P). Free radicals attack cell components and damage cells and tissues of the body. Over time these free radicals are at the root of many diseases and the aging processes. Free radicals are a group of highly reactive substances called oxidants. Free radicals are unavoidable because they are formed during normal metabolic processes that occur in the body. You consume free radicals from some foods and inhale them with air pollution and tobacco smoke. Additionally, free radicals are generated in the environment from radiation and herbicides or pesticides. The scavenger group of vitamins helps intercede, deactivate, and render free radicals harmless before they cause irreversible damage to the body's tissues. Take 3 Deluxe Scavengers daily, divided in doses.

Vitamin E is an antioxidant that accelerates healing and enhances the immune system. Natural Vitamin E (d-Alpha or mixed tocopherol) is 36% more potent than synthetic (dl-Tocopherol), more bioavailable, and better retained. The usual dosage of natural Vitamin E is 800 I.U. daily.

Malic Acid 600 derives from apples and is an important component in the formation of ATP (Adenosine Triphosphate) or cell energy in the body. Malic acid reduces pain and fights fatigue. Use 2 Malic Acid 600 mg, twice per day with meals. If you suffer from fibromyalia, use the Malic Acid Plus instead with Mag Link and/or Mag Chlor. In the *Journal of Nutritional Medicine* studies demonstrated that when malic acid and magnesium (Mag Link or Chlor 85) were given in combination, patients experienced a great deal of relief.

Taurine 1000 is a major inhibitory neurotransmitter amino acid. During times of stress/anxiety, illness, post trauma, depression, or grief, the need for Taurine increases. Studies demonstrate that Taurine controls epileptic seizures, uncontrollable muscular and facial twitches/tics, and aids with hyperactivity. Since Taurine is the major amino acid found in the heart, it plays an important role in smooth heart rhythms. Retinal and eye degeneration occur with Taurine deficiencies. Take 1 Taurine 1000 mg, twice daily.

Arginine is an important amino acid that assists in the urea cycle, which metabolizes nitrogen and proteins. The presence of Arginine in the body stimulates the production of muscle protein synthesis and prevents the breakdown of muscle tissues. Arginine stimulates growth hormone and increases sexual performance. If you have had a problem with herpes in the past, use Arginine with caution and always balance it with 3000 mg of Lysine daily. *Do not use Arginine if you have diabetes, cancer, or schizophrenia.* The usual dosage of Arginine is 1000 mg, twice to three times daily. If you are using Arginine to stimulate growth hormone release, use 2800 to 3000 mg daily, in divided doses.

P5'P (Pyridoxal 5'Phosphate) is the biologically active form of B6. P5'P is safe and effective and you do not have to worry about B6 toxicity. Remember, you must use B6 or P5'P daily to active your amino acids so the body can use them. The usual dose of P5'P is 50 mg daily.

DHEA and Pregnenolone are neurohormones that drop rapidly after the age of 40. Both play an important role in aging and diseases related to aging. DHEA is naturally produced by the adrenal glands. Age, stress, post-trauma, pain, and certain diseases cause your DHEA level to drop dramatically. Studies show DHEA assists with the ability to cope with stress, improves the quality of sleep, and gives more mobility with less joint pain. Before you start taking DHEA or Pregnenolone, it is best to have a DHEA sulfate test drawn, so you know exactly what your level is. After you start taking DHEA or Pregnenolone, repeat the test to see what your level is. If you are over 40, the most common amount of DHEA used is 25 to 50 mg per day upon arising in the morning. If you are taking Hormone Replacement Therapy (HRT), *it is best not to use DHEA or Pregnenolone.*

Pregnenolone is produced in the brain and adrenal gland. Pregnenolone is a direct precursor of DHEA, progesterone, and other steroid hormones. The late researcher and expert on Pregnenolone Dr. Regelson believed that Pregnenolone fights fatigue and is the most potent memory and concentration enhancer available. Take 25 to 100 mg of Pregnenolone per day upon arising in the morning. Monitor your DHEA sulfate level to make sure it remains in the mid-normal range.

Candex is an anti-fungus (yeast) formula. If you have problems with yeast, take 2 capsules upon awakening in the morning, at least one hour before breakfast, and 2 at bedtime, at least two hours after eating, for 30 days. Then for maintenance, take 1 capsule at bedtime.

Curbita is pumpkin seed oil that helps to strengthen the entire bladder system. Use 1 soft gel, twice to three times daily. A deficiency of magnesium can also cause the bladder to spasm.

Olive Leaf Extract (D-Lenolate) is a natural, safe, and effective herb with tremendous healing properties. Research demonstrates that the leaves of the Olive Leaf have exceptional healing power against viruses and bacteria. Olive Leaf extract attacks bacteria directly by strengthening your immune system. D-Lenolate is a patented and the most potent Olive Leaf available. D-Lenolate is Olive Leaf Extract that was used for hospital testing with positive results. D-Lenolate kills viruses, fungus (yeast), bacteria, and parasites. Use 1 to 2 capsules of D-Lenolate, three times daily for 10 days.

Balanced Neurotransmitter Complex + GABA (BNC + GABA) contains the essential and nonessential amino acids and nutrients to produce neurotransmitters in the brain as well as sparking the Krebs cycle or the body's energy producing cycle. Use 1 teaspoon of the powder, twice daily in juice. Note: Use either BNC + GABA or Brain Link; you do not need to use both.

Neurotransmitters underlie every thought and emotion, memory and learning; they carry the signals between all nerves or neurons in the brain. Over half of the 50 neurotransmitters are vital to control post traumatic stress. Remember, drugs only block symptoms, they do not address deficiencies in the brain.

Anxiety and post trauma have a lot of the same symptoms as fear. But it is the uncertainty that lingers long after the stress has lifted and the threat has past that causes the body to release cortisol. The increase of cortisol continues keeps the body in a state of fight-or-flight causing your already stressed adrenals to work harder.

Bibliography

Addiction Science Research and Education Center, University of Texas, College of Pharmacy, 2002.

Appleton, John P., Ed. *The Amygdala.* New York: Wiley-Liss, 1992.

Bechara, A., et al. "Double Dissociation of Conditioning and Declarative Knowledge Relative to the Amygdala and Hippocampus in Humans." Science. 269, 1995, pp. 1115–1118.

Birdsall, Timothy C. "5-Hydroxytryptophan: A Clinically-Effective Serotonin Precursor." *Alternative Medicine Review*, Vol. 3, No. 4, 1998, pp. 271-280.

Blier, P, et al. "Modifications of the Serotonin System by Antidepressant Treatments: Implications fro the Therapeutic Response in Major Depression." *Journal of Clinical Psychopharmacology,* Vol. 7, 1987, pp. 24S–35S.

Breggin, Peter. *Brain Disabling Treatments in Psychiatry.* New York: Springer Publishing Co., 1997.

Calvin, William and George A. Ojemann. *Conversation's with Neil's Brain, The Neural Nature of Thought and Language.* New York: Addison-Wesley Publishing Co., 1994.

Carter, Rita. *Mapping the Mind.* Berkley, CA: University of California Press, 1998.

Cohon, Jay S. *Over Dose.* New York: Jeremy P. Tarcher/Putnam, 2001.

Cooper, Jack R., et al. *The Biochemistry of Neuropharm-acology.* New York: Oxford University Press, 1984???

Davis, Joel. *Endorphins, New Wave of Brain Chemistry.* New York, NY: Wiley, 1982.

Fox, Arnold and Barry Fox. *DLPA To End Chronic Pain and Depression.* New York: Long Shadow Books, 1985.

Gaby, Alan R. *Magnesium.* New Canaan, CT: Keats Publishing, 1994.

Goldstein, Jay. *Betrayal By The Brain.* New York: The Haworth Medical Press, 1996.

Gershon, Michael D. *The Second Brain.* New York: HarperCollin Publishers, 1998.

Glenmullen, Joseph. *Prozac Backlash.* NY: Simon & Schuster, March, 2000.

Holmwood, C., "Chronic Fatigue Syndrome, a Review from the General Practice Perspective." *Australian Family Physician,* Vol. 21, No. 3, March, 1992.

Klatz, Ronald M., ed. *Advances in Anti-Aging Medicine.* Volume 1, Larchmont, NY: Mary Ann Liebert, Inc., 1996.

Kotulak, Ronald. *Inside the Brain.* Kansas City: Andrews and McMeel, 1996.

Klatz, Ronald and Robert Goldman. *Stopping the Clock.* New York: Bantam Books, 1996.

LeDoux, Joseph. "Probing Circuits of Normal and Pathological Fear through Studies of Fear Conditioning." Center for Neuroscience of Fear and Anxiety, Center for Neural Science, New York University, 2002.

LeDoux, Joseph. *Synaptic Self, How Our Brains Become Who We Are.* New York: Penguin Putnam, Inc., 2002.

Leibovitz, Brain. *Carnitine, The Bt Phenomenon.* New York: Bantam Books, 1984.

Lombard, Jay and Carl Germano. *The Brain Wellness Plan.* New York: Kensington Books, 1997.

Milne, Robert, et al. *A Definitive Guide to Headaches.* Tiburon, CA: Future Medicine Publishing, Inc., 1997.

Moyer, Bill. *Healing and the Mind.* New York: Doubleday, 1993.

Murray, Michael. *Boost Your Serotonin Levels, 5-HTP.* New York: Bantam Books, 1998.

Pelletier, Kenneth R. *Mind as Healer, Mind as Slayer.* New York: Delta Trade Books, 1977.

Pert, Candace. *Molecules of Emotion.* New York: Scribner Publishing, 1997.

Pinchot, Roy B. (ed.) *The Brain—Mystery of Matter and Mind.* New York: Torstar Books, Inc., 1984.

Rapp, Doris. *Is This Your Child?* New York: Bantam Books, 1995.

Rately, John J. *A User's Guide to the Brain.* New York: Vintage Books, 2002.

Regelsen, William and Carol Coleman. *The SuperHormone Promise.* New York: Simon & Schuster, 1996.

Restak, Richard M. *Receptors.* New York: Bantam Books, 1994.

Rogers, Sherry. *Pain Free in 6 Weeks.* Sarasota, FL: Sand Key Co, Inc., 2001.

Rogers, Sherry, *Wellness Against All Odds.* Syracuse, NY: Prestige Press, 1994.

"Role of Hormone Testing." *Women's Health Connection.* Vol. 9, No. 1, p. 2.

Sahley, Billie J. *GABA, The Anxiety Amino Acid.* San Antonio: Pain & Stress Publications,® 2001.

Sahley, Billie J. and Katherine M. Birkner. *Heal with Amino Acids.* San Antonio: Pain & Stress Publications,® 2000.

Shaw, D.L., et al. "Management of fatigue: a physiological approach." *American Journal Medical Science,* 1962, pp. 243, 758.

Sinatra, Stephen T. *The CoEnzyme Phenomemon.* Los Angeles. Lowell House, 1998.

Wilson, James L. *Adrenal Fatigue, The 21st Century Stress Syndrome.* Santa Rosa, CA: Health Freedom Nutrition, 2001.

Other Resources

The Anxiety Epidemic by Billie J. Sahley, Ph.D.

The Anti-Depressant Fact Book by Peter R. Breggin, M.D.

Breaking Your Prescribed Addiction by Drs. Billie J. Sahley and K. Birkner

Breaking the Grip of Dangerous Emotions by Dr. Janet Maccaro

Depression Cured at Last by Sherry Rogers, M.D.

Detoxify or Die by Sherry Rogers, M.D.

The E.I. Syndrome by Sherry Rogers, M.D.

Food Allergies Made Simple by Phylis Austin, et al.

GABA, The Anxiety Amino Acid by Billie J. Sahley, Ph.D.

The Great Anxiety Escape by Max Ricketts

Heal with Amino Acids by Drs. Billie Sahley and K. Birkner

Inside the Brain by Ronald Kotulak

Malic Acid And Magnesium For Fibromyalgia and Chronic Pain Syndrome by Dr. Billie J. Sahley

Molecules of Emotion by Candace Pert, Ph.D.

No More Heartburn by Sherry Rogers, M.D.

Overdose (Prescription Drugs and Your Health) by Jay Cohen, M.D.

Pain Free in 6 Weeks by Sherry Rogers, M.D.

Prozac Backlash by Joseph Glenmullen, M.D.

The Second Brain by Michael D. Gershon, M.D.

Tired or Toxic by Sherry Rogers, M.D

Toxic Psychiatry by Peter R. Breggin, M.D.

The Ultimate Nutrient, Glutamine by Judy Shabert, M.D., R.D. and Nancy Ehrlich

Your Drug May Be Your Problem by Peter R. Breggin, M.D.

Index

Other Books by Dr. Billie Sahley

THE ANXIETY EPIDEMIC

How GABA and Other Amino Acids Are The Key To Controlling Anxiety and Panic Attacks

Billie Jay Sahley, Ph.D.

HEAL With AMINO ACIDS and Nutrients

Billie J. Sahley, Ph.D.
Kathy Birkner, C.R.N.A., Ph.D.

GABA
The *Anxiety* Amino Acid

Revolutionary Discoveries of How GABA Affects Mind, Mood, Memory, and Behavior

Billie Jay Sahley, Ph.D.
Author of The Anxiety Epidemic

CONTROL HYPERACTIVITY A.D.D. NATURALLY

Breakthrough Information About Amino Acid and Vitamin Therapy That Can Change Your Child's Life!

Billie J. Sahley, Ph.D.
Author of Is Ritalin Necessary?

Is RITALIN *Necessary?*
THE RITALIN

Why Ritalin And Other Drugs Are NOT The Answer To A.D.D./A.D.H.D. Amino Acids Offer Safe, Effective Natural Alternatives

Billie J. Sahley, Ph.D.
Author of Control Hyperactivity A.D.D. Naturally

BREAKING YOUR *PRESCRIBED* ADDICTION

A Guide to Coming Off Tranquilizers, Antidepressants, Pain Pills, and More Using Amino Acids & Nutrients

Billie J. Sahley, Ph.D.
Kathy Birkner, C.R.N.A., Ph.D.

Malic Acid and Magnesium for Fibromyalgia and Chronic Pain Syndrome

Understand Why You Hurt All Over And What You Can Take Naturally To Stop The Pain

Billie J. Sahley, Ph.D., C.N.C.
Author of Is Ritalin Necessary?

To Order Call 1-800-669-2256 or go to

THE MELATONIN REPORT

How Melatonin Protects Your Brain and Body Functions . . . Sleep - Wake Cycle Seasonal Affective Disorder and More

Billie J. Sahley, Ph.D.

http://www.painstresscenter.com

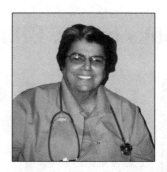

About the Author

Billie J. Sahley, Ph.D., is Executive Director of the Pain & Stress Center in San Antonio. She is a Board Certified Medical Psychotherapist & Psychodiagnostician, Behavior Therapist, and an Orthomolecular Therapist. She is a Diplomate in the American Academy of Pain Management. Dr. Sahley is a graduate of the University of Texas, Clayton University School of Behavioral Medicine, and U.C.L.A. School of Integral Medicine. She is also a Certified Nutritional Consultant (C.N.C.). Additionally, she has studied advanced nutritional biochemistry through Jeffrey Bland, Ph.D. at Institute of Functional Medicine. She is a member of the Huxley Foundation/Academy of Orthomolecular Medicine, Academy of Psychosomatic Medicine, North American Nutrition and Preventive Medicine Association. In addition, she holds memberships in the Sports Medicine Foundation, American Association of Hypnotherapists, and American Mental Health Counselors Association. She also sits on the Scientific and Medical Advisory Board for Inter-Cal Corporation.

Dr. Sahley wrote: *The Anxiety Epidemic*; *Control Hyperactivity/ A.D.D. Naturally; GABA, the Anxiety Amino Acid; Post Trauma and Chronic Emotional Fatigue; The Melatonin Report; Is Ritalin Necessary? The Ritalin Report;* and has recorded numerous audiocassette tapes. She coauthored *Breaking Your Prescribed Addiction* and *Heal With Amino Acids*.

In addition, Dr. Sahley holds three U.S. patents for: SAF, Calms Kids (SAF For Kids), and Anxiety Control 24. Dr. Sahley devotes the majority of her time to research, writing, and development of natural products to address brain deficiencies.